TOP 15 HEALTH AND FITNESS TIPS

- Improve Your Health Status

KANHA GUPTA

ISBN: 9798537965473

DEDICATION

To lovers of books....

I hope this book helps you to get your health to a better level, that it allows you to stir the hearts and minds of many, many people.

I would love nothing more than to see your book in the hands of people everywhere – readers walking down the street, browsers in the bookstores, vacationers at the beach, students in the classroom, secretaries at the office, mothers at home.

That's a great challenge, and may be it's not possible to achieve. But it is certainly worth an attempt. Even several attempts.

Take your time. Do it right. Focus on your health. Be happy and enjoy.

That's the best advice I can give you.

CONTENTS

ACKNOWLEDGEMENT

First and foremost, I would like you thank God for his never-ending grace, mercy and provision during what ended up being one of the toughest times of my life. I would also like to thank my astoundingly supportive parents, there should be no "hope" without any of you. Last but not the least, I would also like to thank my brilliant and truly outstanding friends whose visions steered this work from day one.

For those who have touched my life in any way since I've started in this book, you all know who you are, and I truly grateful for all you have done.

1.

Doing Dead Lift Exercises - The Proper Way

Individuals who need to enhance their power, posture, and universal fitness typically encompass useless raise sporting events of their health software. This exercising is an indispensable element of a power improvement software that truly works each muscle withinside the frame and emphasizes hips, thighs, buttocks, decrease returned, the shoulders, and the forearms. These frame components are the postural chain of the frame and are vital for retaining right posture. The useless raise is taught via way of means of health professionals to those who need to growth their stage of power and muscle mass. The useless raise is one of the high-quality sporting events for enhancing one's physique, particularly if that health aim desires to be attained in only a quick length of time. The high-quality issue approximately this exercising is that it does now no longer require any fancy devices and equipment. All one wishes is a barbell and a flat surface. The barbell may be loaded with as tons weight as it is easy to take care of and choose it off the floor whilst preserving the returned straight. The useless raise additionally has feasible rehabilitation benefits. Research has proven that the mild to excessive hamstring interest executed as a part of a useless raise ordinary can also additionally assist support the Anterior Cruciate Ligament in the course of rehabilitation. The motion of this exercising interprets nicely into actual existence due to the fact it may be likened to bending and lifting. However, unsupervised and wrong execution of useless lifts can also additionally motive injury. It is critical to seek advice from a physician earlier than undertaking excessive depth sporting events just like the useless raise. Individuals who revel in returned ache and different muscle aches due to excessive depth exercising can also additionally take Food and Drug Administration (FDA) permitted ache relievers like Tramadol. Tramadol is a artificial ache reliever that has received the approval of the Food and Drug Administration (FDA). It works via way of means of binding the receptors of the mind which can be accountable for transmitting painful sensations at some stage in the frame. The use of this drug blended with bodily remedy hurries up the healing manner and restores everyday bodily interest. Several scientific research display that this medicine has a low abuse fee as compared to different ache relievers. In addition, Tramadol facet outcomes are milder as compared to different ache relieving tablets out withinside the market. These facet outcomes can also additionally encompass nausea, constipation, dizziness, headache, drowsiness, and vomitting. Individuals have to seek advice from their docs earlier than taking this medicine. Though Tramadol facet outcomes are moderate and bearable, it is able to now no longer be utilized by people with positive fitness situations and scientific history. This drug may engage with different tablets which can also additionally result in improvement of greater undesirable facet outcomes. Prevention is higher than cure. Rather than searching for scientific interest to deal with injuries, this circumstance may be avoided nicely undertaking weight lifting and different varieties of exercising. A physician-permitted health software which incorporates flexibility training, warm-up, and funky down sporting events can also additionally reduce the improvement of injuries. If this stuff fails, ask your physician approximately Tramadol.

2.
Links Between Stress Shift Work & Serotonin Levels

The twenty first Century is quality characterised through the arrival of ultra-current technology, international industrial and commercial enterprise, and the unstoppable preference to get and live ahead. Because of those factors, commercial enterprise groups compete in a global wherein the financial system is lively 24 hours a day, seven days a week. This phenomenon created a call for for personnel that might paintings even throughout the night time upto the wee hours of the morning. This paintings time table reversed worker lifestyle, making the day their time to for sleeping. Shifts might also additionally disrupt the everyday frame features, bog down sleep cycles, and decrease the frame's serotonin stages. Serotonin is a neurotransmitter this is observed withinside the principal frightened machine and influences a couple of features like mood, sleep, sexuality, and appetite. This neurotransmitter may additionally sell mobileular regeneration. Studies display that non-day shift people have a tendency to have decrease stages of "feel-good" hormones known as serotonin. Researchers on the University of Buenos Aires led through Dr. Carlos J, Pirola studied 683 guys and as compared 437 days people to 246 shift people. The results, the shift people' serotonin stages, measured via blood assessments had been considerably decrease than the ones on normal day schedules. In addition to decreased serotonin stages, shift people had been additionally observed to have better cholesterol, hip-to-waist ratios, multiplied blood strain, and better triglyceride stages. Because serotonin stages administer sleep styles and different frame features, the University of Buenos Aires look at advised that shift paintings may additionally cause a so-known as Shift Work Sleep Disorder. People with this disease have a tendency to stay wakeful once they ought to be sleeping. These people may be very worn-out throughout waking hours. This disease takes area due to a piece time table that takes area throughout the everyday sleep period. Because of this, humans who've problem getting sleep due to the fact that their bodies are nonetheless programmed to be wakeful. The time of being asleep and being wakeful isn't like what the frame's inner clock expects. Other research additionally observed out that non-general and night time shift paintings might also additionally have an effect on the cardiovascular and metabolic systems. These research advocate that there's a opportunity that shift paintings is at once answerable for excessive blood strain and multiplied frame fat, in accordance the researchers of the Buenos Aires look at. In addition to the disruption of sleep styles, decreased stages of serotonin also are related to different situations like stress, anxiety, and depression. Lifestyle modifications can cause progressed serotonin stages. To make serotonin stages constant, sleep styles ought to be constant and meals regimens ought to consist of vital nutrients and minerals to govern the serotonin stages. Certain capsules and materials like caffeine, nicotine, alcohol, and antidepressants ought to be averted due to the fact they'll dissipate serotonin production. Individuals who need to enhance their serotonin stages can use medicinal drug to useful resource them of their goal. The amino acid 5-HTP may be taken as a complement and enhance the frame's capacity to fabricate serotonin. Another amino acid known as L-tryptophan is utilized by the frame to provide serotonin. However, earlier than taking those supplements, sufferers are cautioned to are looking for the approval of docs and different fitness professionals. Individuals who select to paintings withinside the night time ought to hold good enough relaxation to reduce ill-results that can develop. Healthy life and nutritious meals regimens might also additionally enhance serotonin stages and enhance one's best of life.

3.

Seven Tips For A Long And Healthy Life

As proper as present day, scientific generation is, it could in no way prevent from the troubles because of an existence fashion this is unhealthy. Instead of having a present day scientific restore for each problem, it's far some distance higher to stay in this sort of manner that you'll not often fall ill. An ounce of prevention is honestly higher than a pound of cure. Here are seven suggestions on the way to stay an extended and wholesome existence. In addition, the identical existence fashion that lets you keep away from contamination additionally lets you lose weight.

a. Get Enough Exercise

In the beyond humans needed to use their bodily our bodies withinside the path in their ordinary paintings. But nowadays a person might also additionally arise, visit paintings in a vehicle, then take a seat down, arise to move domestic withinside the vehicle and while arriving at domestic, take a seat down down once more for the relaxation of the day. In this sort of existence there's no bodily labor. This bodily state of being inactive is one of the primary motives for a number of sicknesses. Sport, running on foot and different matters ought to be introduced to our existence if our ordinary paintings does now no longer require us to exert ourselves physically.

b. Go to sleep whilst you sense sleepy

This might also additionally sound easy, however many humans live up overdue even if their frame is telling them that it's time to sleep. Yoga and Ayurvedic docs additionally say that it's far higher to sleep withinside the night time and be energetic at some point of the day. However, humans together with college students will take espresso and stimulants to examine overdue into the night time. Others increase the addiction of last energetic at night time and slumbering at some point of the day. While we are able to do this, it finally takes a toll on fitness. Alternative fitness docs say that this type of unnatural residing is one of the contributing elements withinside the causation of most cancers and different sicknesses.

c. Eat whilst you sense hungry

This is likewise an easy idea, however all over again we regularly pass in opposition to the messages of the frame. If you devour out of addiction or because of social stress at sure time of the day, even if you have no actual urge for food, then you'll now no longer digest your meals properly. Acidity and indigestion begin, and this contributes to the chance of different extra complicated sicknesses taking root. Having an urge for food is without a doubt a signal of proper fitness, however when you have no urge for food you need to wait a chunk after which devour. (If you haven't any urge for food even after expecting an affordable quantity of time, then you definitely need to seek advice from a medical doctor due to the fact something is wrong).

<u>d. Fast on a Regular, Systematic Basis</u>

If you'll ask any man or woman to paintings three hundred and sixty-five days in step with yr with none relaxation, they could bitch and say that they ought to have a few relaxation in any other case they'll damage down. But we've got in no way stricken to invite or to reflect on consideration on our digestive organs which we compel to paintings day by day without a relaxation. They can't protest the manner someone could to his boss, however they do provide us indicators that they can't paintings non-stop. When we forget about the ones indicators and nonetheless compel them to paintings, the ones organs damage down. That is why periodic fasting is necessary. Refrain from consuming for one whole day. This offers a relaxation on your digestive organs and additionally facilitates withinside the removal of wastes out of your frame. Regular fasting lets in someone to benefit more time for highbrow or religious pursuits. Fasting isn't always for hermits in a cave, however is a realistic exercise that absolutely everyone can exercise.

<u>e. Wash with cool water earlier than going to bed</u>

As cited above, right sleep is crucial for the upkeep of fitness. If you wash your crucial motor and sensory organs (hands, arms, eyes, legs, mouth, genitals) earlier than sleep the usage of cool water, this can loosen up you and put together you for deep sleep.

f. Perform meditation on a normal basis

Your frame is related on your mind. Many of the sicknesses of this period are psychosomatic. Stress and tension take their toll on our bodily fitness. Meditation is an intellectual exercising which, amongst different matters, lets in you to detach yourself from the issues of existence. Learn an easy approach and do it regularly.

g. Get up early each day

Once more the vintage proverb, "Early to bed, early to upward thrust makes someone wholesome, rich and wise." I don't understand if it's going to make you rich, however it's going to honestly make you wholesome. Your frame wishes simply sufficient sleep, now no longer an excessive amount of and now no longer too little.

Follow those suggestions and also you can't pass wrong.

4.
Life Advice Looking Through A Window

Living in today's metropolitan international of cell phones, cellular computer systems and different high-tech devices isn't simply irritating however very impersonal. We make cash after which make investments our effort and time in making extra cash. Does it end? Not typically due to the fact we're in no way satisfied. How in many instances have we satisfied ourselves that if simplest we had a few extra cash, existence could be so sweet? But then, after receiving a large raise, we recognise that it wasn't sufficient and that we want extra?

What Should You Do?

I actually have examined many books on existence along with Robin Sharma's Monk says this and the monk says that, and all of them appear to mention that cash isn't necessary. But it is. Can you do without coins and quite a few it? I understand I can't. So, I went to the neighbourhood Rabbi and requested for recommendation so that it will assist me locate my genuine manner in existence. The rabbi nodded and took me to the window. "What do you spot?" he requested me. Promptly, I answered, "I can see human beings on foot back and forth and a blind guy is begging for alms on the left corner." The Rabbi nodded and guided me to a huge reflect. "Now appearance and inform me what you spot?" "I can see myself," I guy answered. The Rabbi smiled. "Now you couldn't see all people else. The reflect and the window are each constituted of the equal uncooked material: glass, however due to the fact on certainly considered one among them they have got implemented a skinny layer of silver, while you study all of it you could see is your very own reflection." The Rabbi positioned his arm on my shoulders. "Compare yourself to the ones portions of glass. Without the silver layer, you noticed the opposite human beings and felt compassion for them. When you're protected with silver, you spot simplest yourself." I checked out the Rabbi and stared. "I don't understand." The Rabbi continued. "You turn into a person simplest if have the braveness to cast off the silver masking over your eyes for you to once more see and love others." He patted me on my returned and despatched me on my manner. I actually have notion of what he stated and are available to the belief that he had a point. Yes. We want cash and we need to no longer goal to steer a moneyless existence; it is useless and could simplest reason us and our households many heartbreaks withinside the future.

Instead, I advise that we need to observe the recommendation the Rabbi gave me. When we method existence thru a silver masking, all we're capable of see is ourselves. But discard that masking, and you may be capable of see and experience every person else.

In existence, we're allowed to and need to be capable of study each type of mirrors, however we need to consider that a reflect displays simplest us; a window is the door to compassion, fitness and genuine wealth. In different words, are seeking for wealth through all means, however don't allow it dissuade you from existence, human beings, youngsters and the negative and needy.

5.
How Anabolic Steroids Came To Humans

It becomes withinside the past due Nineteen Thirties while the substances, popularly referred to as anabolic steroids had been first evolved for the remedy of hypogonadism, that is incompetence of the gonads, mainly because of low manufacturing of testosterone in males. Hypogonadism is the situation wherein male testes do now no longer produce enough testosterone for regular boom, improvement, and sexual functioning. It consequence in poor improvement of secondary intercourse traits and in prepubertal males, a frame with lengthy legs and a quick trunk. Anabolic steroids had been ordinarily produced for clinical use. They had been to start with used to deal with behind schedule puberty, and a few kinds of impotence. Later, many scientists accomplishing research on anabolic steroids discovered that those steroids may want to facilitate the boom of skeletal muscle tissue in laboratory animals. The research brought about using anabolic steroids withinside the remedy of losing of the frame because of HIV contamination or numerous different diseases. However, the boom triggering assets of anabolic steroids additionally brought about abuse of anabolic steroids via way of means of bodybuilders, weightlifters, athletes, and jocks in different sports. Anabolic steroids are one of the maximum famous in addition to one of the maximum arguable capsules today. They are to be had in numerous manufacturers at the market. Anabolic steroids are to be had as oral anabolic steroids, injectable anabolic steroids, and anabolic steroid gels or creams. These capsules are generally taken withinside the sample known as CYCLING, this means that taking doses of anabolic steroids over a selected duration of time, preventing for a duration, and beginning again. Anabolic steroids are utilized in stacks, and this manner of the use of steroids is known as STACKING, this means that the use of anabolic steroids combining specific kinds of steroids. Often anabolic steroids are utilized in stacks via way of means of bodybuilders or different energy jocks. The customers accept as true with that stacking anabolic steroids assist to provide an impact on muscle length this is more than the outcomes of the use of every drug individually. Another famous manner of the use of anabolic steroids is PYRAMIDING, that is the manner wherein steroid customers step up using steroids slowly. They boom the quantity of medicine used at one time and/or the dose and frequency of 1 or extra steroids, accomplishing the very best quantity at mid-cycle and slowly narrowing the dose towards the quits of the cycle.

<u>6.</u>
<u>How A Natural Enzyme Can Improve And Maintain Your Health</u>

Over thirty years ago, a German physician, Dr. Hans Neiper, confronted with the troubles which might be nevertheless unresolved via way of means of mainstream medicinal drug today, appeared to nature to discover a manner that could cope with all and any kind of infection. Inflammation is something withinside the frame that must now no longer be there. Any "non dwelling tissue". And pretty simply, that is pretty much something that reasons pain. Blockages, consisting of withinside the head or chest from mucus, like catarrh, sinus or bronchial troubles, asthma, emphysema, or industrially brought about troubles which includes asbestosis. Things like blood clots, prostate troubles, arthritis, ulcers and a mass of different troubles that your medical doctor will let you know can't be helped are all because of infection. Serrapeptase is the enzyme that the silkworm makes use of to dissolve its cocoon. Dr. Neiper realised that if the silkworm, while it turns from being the computer virus right into a moth, and it does so in a completely quick time, should have something that dissolves "non dwelling tissue", due to the fact the cocoon is a tough shape of lifeless tissue. Dr. Neiper separated the enzyme out, gave it to his sufferers and finished magnificent results, very quickly. He gave it to at least one affected person due for amputation of a hand due to a blocked artery. It cleared the blockage and the person stored his hand. He additionally pronounced that Serrapeptase dissolved blood clots and brought about varicose veins to reduce or diminish. To gain the big quantity required withinside the global today, Serrapeptase is now obviously processed commercially thru fermentation. Histological research has found out the effective anti-inflammatory results of this obviously taking place enzyme. Known viable advantages can be the resolving of pain; handling lung troubles; eye troubles; ENT troubles (Ear-Nose-Throat); trauma; infection of any kind; cardiovascular problems and really importantly, arthritis. In 25 years of being prescribed via way of means of German medical doctors, no dangerous facet results were pronounced. Serrapeptase can, and does, solve many troubles that medical doctors inform us are insoluble. However, we want to recollect that a few of the troubles we revel in with our fitness are frequently intently tied to our diet. If we consume junk meals, we are able to get junk fitness. When buying withinside the supermarket, have a take a observe the labels. How many E numbers or matters which might be sincerely now no longer proper, herbal meals are there withinside the packet? Also, something this is withinside the shape of so called "sugar free" continuously consists of aspartame and different matters which might be unfavourable to our fitness. So, attempt to preserve to a very good diet. Alternative remedies, a lot of that have stood the check of time, in a few instances many masses of years, sooner or later provide wish to quite a few people. Serrapeptase is a latest addition to the list, being "discovered" most effective 35 or so years ago. But it's miles one which works for lots of people.

7.
Prostate Health Learn The Basics

It may be irritating and perplexing to discover what truely works for a man's prostate fitness. In this newsletter I've summarized a number of the essential pointers and guidelines you must know. And if you've observed something that has truely labored for you, that you have demonstrated thru trial and observation, please allow me know. I'd like that allows you to proportion it with others. First, examine the subsequent listing of useful guidelines associated with progressed prostate fitness and benign prostate enlargement.

a. Urinary tract infections (UTI's) are frequently associated with an enlarged prostate. Candida and infections like prostatitis also are related. Candida is a not unusualplace and insidious situation you must make certain to eliminate. At my internet site I even have a easy self-check for candida.

b. Do pelvic physical games to boom move through tightening your pelvic muscle groups deliberately at the least one hundred instances a day. Raise your attention of the internal global of your pelvic area. Give separate attention for your buttocks, decrease abdominals, scrotum, urethra, and sphincter.

c. Use Prosperon to elevate your testosterone degree naturally.

d. Drink lots of water, each day, to flush out your system.

e. Move to a low animal-protein and grain-wealthy diet, or a few variants at the macrobiotic.

f. Keep your weight in check.

g. Keep a magazine so one can tune and recognize, as quickly as possible, what's running for you, and what's now no longer. Think approximately your signs and symptoms for yourself; don't simply rely upon your doctor!

h. Realize that hormones are hormones and nutrients are nutrients. When his PSA check effects have been too high, a pal determined to heal himself through doing an anti-parasite treatment. It did not harm, however your prostate has to do with hormones, and wishes to be treated in this degree. You can't position sparkling oil on your automobile while you're out of fueloline after which marvel why your engine won't work!

i. Visualize that you are in a good deal with health and that your prostate and urethra features well. Approach your frame with love, as it's miles a part of your temple wherein the soul resides.

Melatonin: A wonderful examine completed at Tel Aviv University confirmed that the melatonin receptors withinside the prostate may want to suppress prostate enlargement.

Researchers observed that an enlarged prostate is because of the imbalance of estrogen and testosterone that takes place as we age. They in addition cited that the extra estrogen additionally interferes with the ordinary metabolism of melatonin (J. Clin. Endoc. Metab. 82 (1997) p. 2535 – 41).

Their recommendation then, is to take 1-three mg. of melatonin complement each night. (Stick with this dosage; as with maximum medicines, greater is in no way better.) Take it ONLY within side the darkness of night, so as now no longer to intrude with the frame's herbal manufacturing of melatonin earlier than sunrise. Go to mattress through ten o'clock additionally, to get a terrific night's rest.

8.
Dealing With Death Anxiety

The worry of demise is one of the oldest fears of the human race, stemming in large part from the reality that no one is totally certain what's "on the alternative facet." On a few instances, the worry of demise will become even worse whilst the man or woman is tormented by a terminal infection and is necessarily conscious that his time is nearly up. This feeling, now and again noted as "demise anxiety" is regularly observed via way of means of bouts of melancholy and revel in some of troubles linked to their interpersonal relationships. This "demise anxiety" can now and again be a trouble for the human beings across the death, though a few mental facet results have additionally been observed.

For the maximum part, this trouble is basically unnoticed in want of both prolonging the affected person's life, or making their remaining days as snug and painless as viable. For maximum clinical professionals, the bodily thing of demise is some distance less difficult to cope with than the emotional and mental aspects of it. However, pretty recently, increasingly more human beings are beginning to take note of the troubles posed via way of means of "demise anxiety" and the measures that might be taken to assist lessen the emotional ache of these involved. Inevitably, this consists of each the death affected person himself and the human beings round him, who could must cope with the emotional reckoning even after the affected person has handed away.

The melancholy that someone can experience due to the fact of "demise anxiety" isn't any less complicated to cope with than normal melancholy could be. In reality, because the inevitability of demise is looming over the horizon, it's far pretty viable that the trouble could surely be worse than normal. This is proper for each the affected person and the affected person's cherished ones, who could must additionally cope with the awful truth that a person they care approximately goes to die. When taken into context, the melancholy should effortlessly be visible as something this is compounding even past demise, such that a trouble that simplest severely affected the affected person "infects" the human beings the affected person left behind.

Recent findings display that assist companies had been regularly desirable for assisting human beings emotionally put together for demise. This is for each sufferer and the sufferers' families, who all may want only a little more assist to address the appearance of demise. Others locate it useful to be uncovered to others who're suffering, or have suffered through, the equal troubles. Most psychologists consider that being uncovered to others that experience the equal pressures and troubles may be instrumental in assisting a person address each the lack of a cherished one and the capability mental harm that a terminal infection can do.

Standard assist materials, consisting of magazines, pamphlets, and the like, were in flow a few of the terminally sick for some years now. Most intellectual fitness professional word that those do have an observable effective impact on someone's typical temper throughout intervals of "demise anxiety," however they regularly aren't enough to preserve a person from slinking into melancholy. These may be useful and are generally observed without problems withinside the workplaces of medical doctors and professionals who often cope with this form of trouble.

<u>9.</u>
<u>A Guide To A Better Mental Health</u>

While absolutely fictional, the enigmatic idea knowns as "The Force" is primarily based totally on a few very actual concepts. In the movie, Star Wars, the "Force" is frequently spoken of with the aid of using participants of a spiritual order referred to as the Jedi. The warrior-clergymen of the Jedi Order served as the primary proponents of what they believed to be the middle ideas of The Force. The idea and the order are fictional, however the concepts with the aid of using which the Jedi lived their lives are remarkable publications to residing one's lifestyles, specially amidst all of the chaos of the today's world. For so long as the "Dark Side" of The Force is equated now no longer to evil however to poor impacts in one's lifestyles, the concepts of the Jedi Code can effortlessly be used to shape a non-public philosophy for residing a great lifestyle, entire with a wholesome intellectual attitude. Below you'll discover the middle concepts of the Jedi philosophy, and a few thoughts on how they may be tailored to the rigors and tribulations of today's lifestyles. There isn't any emotion; there's peace. Being capable of manipulate one's feelings became vital to a Jedi, as their obligations frequently required that they stay as goal as possible. Fear and tension could have poor outcomes on one's decision-making, which in flip can wreak havoc on one's lifestyles. By taking manipulate of one's strain and tension, keeping apart it from the obligations that want to be done, you could correctly discover higher answers in your troubles than you'll have in case you permit your tension have an effect on your evaluation of the situation. This idea does now no longer suggest denying one's feelings, because doing so can bring about greater tension issues and mental problems than it solves. It simply says that humans must permit common sense and evaluation manual their selections, now no longer their feelings. There isn't anyt any ignorance; there's understanding. The Jedi Order espoused the decided pursuit of understanding. To help the hunt for enlightenment, they constructed a grand library that contained volumes of facts on diverse subjects and disciplines that have been vital to train and educate a Jedi. They additionally shared that understanding, to higher enlighten the identical humans they have been trying to protect. Many troubles with tension and phobias may be alleviated if humans simply took the time to apprehend things. A little understanding can assist a person conquer the worry and tension that one encounters while uncovered to a completely alien culture. In a few cases, tension issues can also be tackled sincerely with the aid of using equipping one's thoughts with enough understanding approximately the supply of the tension, consequently permitting someone to higher apprehend and face the problem. There isn't any ardour; there's serenity. Similar to the primary principle, the Jedi believed that being too enthusiastic about something became dangerous, as it is able to cloud one's judgment and objectivity. For humans of their position, objectivity became vital in almost all situations. The identical may be stated of quite a good deal everybody withinside the today's world. Emotions and ardour can cloud our cappotential to make properly selections, in addition to have a destructive impact on our cappotential to apprehend our errors and accurate them to avoid similarly damage. Being calm amidst the face of a not possible forms can cross an extended manner to maintaining one's kingdom of intellectual fitness strong and some distance away from "going postal." As lengthy as you don't permit your strain and tension increase with the aid of using living at the poor, then your thoughts are serene and you could then make higher selections and take a clearer examine what goes on in one's lifestyles. There isn't anyt any demise, there's best The Force. The Jedi believed that once a person dies, they grow to be one with The Force. This allowed them to look demise now no longer as a poor event, however simply a transition that one became unavoidably going to get past. Adapting this to fashionable lifestyles, poor activities may be portrayed as the "demise" the philosophy mentions, with "The Force" appearing as a metaphor for lifestyles itself. In different words, it is essentially declaring that, irrespective of all of the poor activities in one's lifestyles, irrespective of all of the worry and tension, the nausea prompted with the aid of using company and familial duties, there's nevertheless lifestyles itself. To use one metaphor to give an explanation for another, if something horrific comes your manner, make an effort out to prevent and smell the roses. Your whole lifestyles will now no longer be dictated with the aid of using one vehicle crash or an unfair termination. Life is going on and actions on, and so must you. Taking all the above concepts into account, it's miles hard to look how they may fail to cause a higher kingdom of thoughts, even amidst the chaos of today's lifestyles. That is, if they may be observed like a non-public philosophy and now no longer taken as mere guidelines. Besides, if one espouses the alternative of the above concepts, one is susceptible to burn out as an alternative quickly.

10.
Five Ways To Manage Your Diets For Diabetes

Since my analysis with diabetes on the age of eleven, my personal eating regimen has modified dramatically. I hold my modern healthful weight with a wonderful eating regimen/ingesting plan. If you do plan on dropping greater than approximately a stone in weight then I could go to your health practitioner for greater pointers on a way to do that without risk.

I've had diabetes for seven years now, however to inform you that how I hold weight is best could be absolutely incorrect of me. However, I can suggest you to comply with my steps due to the fact I recognize what works and what doesn't. Before I surely start I have to additionally say that I had been delivered up via way of means of wonderful dad and mom who taught me to consume the entirety, and so I do! If there may be some thing which you don't like, there are hundreds of different diabetic recipes and thoughts that you may consume and appreciate.

I am a college scholar and I like to shop for sparkling and natural produce from wherein I live. I trust that that is essential due to the fact it is able to be the maximum precise in your frame and comprise greater vitamins and nutrients than maximum grocery store produce. I want to supply meals from my fortnightly farmers marketplace in town, which sells first rate meat and dairy produce and sparkling in season fruit and greens. This is some other essential element to bear in mind, that ingesting fruit and greens of their season method that they may flavor higher in addition to doing you precise.

I even have a variety of affect from Western European cuisine (specifically France and Italy) as you may tell, however I do now no longer profess to be a chef and the entirety is simple to make and really convenient. I even have examine infinite eating regimen books and diabetic recipe/eating regimen books, and I got here to a end that I assume surely works. I fused all the good stuff from the diets (however now no longer from each eating regimen) and form of prepare my personal one. I name this my Juvenile Diabetes Healthy Diet!

The "rules" that I could lay down are as follows:

<u>a. Cut returned on snacks after which alternate the sort of snacks you consume.</u>
Certainly my largest downfall even though it wasn't surely obvious to me. When I first began out at University, I had very little habitual which supposed that filling my day become tough and popping into the kitchen for a snack, irrespective of how healthful it felt, become a everyday occurence. This is one of the toughest activities for a few human beings, however organising a wonderful habitual is critical to wonderful diabetes care. The sorts of snacks to be ingesting are unsalted nuts, dried unsweetened fruit, sparkling fruit, sparkling greens (I love

sparkling pink pepper and cucumber), darkish chocolate (richer and nicer and also you handiest need 2 squares usually).

<u>b. Cut returned on white flour and embody wholemeal carbs.</u>
This is the maximum critical a part of your eating regimen, and the element that may display the largest growth in lack of weight. Some diets in truth jsut attention in this point, and are very successful. Wholemeal (in particular stoneground wholemeal) is so precise for you and has a lot greater flavour in it that switching is plenty less difficult than you assume. Most human beings are surely amazed on the levels you may get in you grocery store, once more bear in mind that the bread this is fine for you is the only this is hottest with least perservatives or delivered ingredients. Also, brown or basmati rice is wonderful with a adorable nutty texture. Wholemeal pasta is wonderful and in your potatoes I could absolutely advocate the smaller new potatoes.

<u>c. Stop consuming cocktails, begin consuming wine.</u>
Cocktails are complete of sugar, colourants and preservatives. As a scholar I even have had hundreds of exercise at going out and now no longer consuming cocktails, so my drink of preference is Malibu and Diet Coke if I sense I should drink some thing and I make it final all night. I can then pinnacle up with Diet Coke (which has nearly no sugar in it) and it seems as aleven though I am consuming Malibu, who's to recognize. If

you're out at a restaurant, pink wine is plenty higher than something else you may order, (besides water of course!) and it's been confirmed that the anti-oxidants in pink wine are wonderful for maintaining a healthful heart. The endorsed quantity is one glass an afternoon together along with your nighttime meal.

4. Start cooking **greater fruit and greens.**

Fresh fruit and greens are a wonderful manner to get all of the nutrients and minerals you need. And there are such a lot of exclusive approaches wherein to prepare dinner dinner greens, however I locate that uncooked is the fine accompanied intently via way of means of steamed. Both of those approaches keep all their herbal goodness as nicely. I will comply with this submit with some other diabetes recipes submit.

5. Drink **more water.**

I recognize you've got got heard human beings say this frequently before, however the advantages of consuming greater water are endless. A few pointers on a way to get greater water into your day are first off to place bottles of water at all of the locations you pass withinside the residence or work. So preserve one to your desk, for your desk, a pitcher withinside the kitchen, the bedroom, the sitting room, etc. Try and drink these kind of glasses up and you'll be nicely for your manner to eight glasses an afternoon. The trick is to feature a pitcher each few days or so, in case you attempt to drink all that water in a single pass you won't be so willing to drink eight glasses once more, accept as true with me! Have a pass, it's first rate how wonderful you may sense.

11.

New Program Helps Children With Attention Deficit Hyperactivity Disorder (ADHD)

Studies display that interest deficit hyperactivity disease (ADHD) stays a hassle with adolescents withinside the U.S.

According to a look at via way of means of the Mayo Foundation for Medical Education and Research, 75 percentage of kids are recognized with ADHD via way of means of age 19. Those laid low with the disease are much more likely to enjoy studying troubles in regions including studying and writing.

Many of those problems are because of troubles with decoding, comprehension and retention. Some symptoms and symptoms that a toddler is having hassle with those responsibilities are as follows:

* Having troubles sounding out phrases and spotting phrases which are out of context.
* Reading orally at a slower fee than maximum kids of the identical age.
* Confusing the meanings of phrases and sentences.
* Showing problem in distinguishing extensive facts from minor details.
* Having hassle remembering or summarizing what's read.

Fortunately, there's wish for kids with ADHD who're having hassle studying and writing. For many, the solution lies in looking films, including those evolved via way of means of SFK

Media Specially for Kids Corp.

ReadENT studying gadget is a patented application that uses "Reading Movies" to assist kids with unique training desires expand studying and language competencies whilst being entertained.

These films use an modern device called "Action Captions" that indicates spoken phrases on display screen in actual time, with out disrupting the go with the drift of the movie. By presenting those visible phrases, the films make it less complicated for visitors to comprehend language principles and construct vocabulary.

ReadENT Reading Movies are to be had as interactive DVDs of the traditional kids's films "20,000 Leagues Under the Sea," "Tales of Gulliver's Travels" and "The Trojan Horse." They additionally include interactive video games and quizzes to make the studying enjoy even greater fun.

12.
All About Personality Disorders

Question :-

Many of the signs and symptoms and symptoms and symptoms which you describe observe to different character problems as well (for instance, the histrionic, the delinquent and the borderline character problems). Are we to assume that every one character problems are interrelated?

Answer :-

The type of Axis II character problems – deeply ingrained, maladaptive, lifelong conduct styles – withinside the Diagnostic and Statistical Manual, fourth edition, textual content revision [American Psychiatric Association. DSM-IV-TR, Washington, 2000] – or the DSM-IV-TR for short – has come below sustained and extreme complaint from its inception in 1952.

The DSM IV-TR adopts a specific method, postulating that character problems are "qualitatively awesome medical syndromes" (p. 689). This is broadly doubted. Even the difference made among "regular" and "disordered" personalities is an increasing number of being rejected. The "diagnostic thresholds" among regular and bizarre are both absent or weakly supported.

The polythetic shape of the DSM's Diagnostic Criteria – best a subset of the standards is good enough grounds for a diagnosis – generates unacceptable diagnostic heterogeneity.

In different words, humans identified with the identical character sickness may also proportion best one criterion or none.

The DSM fails to make clear the precise courting among Axis II and Axis I problems and the manner persistent youth and developmental issues have interaction with character problems.

The differential diagnoses are indistinct and the character problems are insufficiently demarcated. The end result is immoderate co-morbidity (a couple of Axis II diagnoses).

The DSM incorporates little dialogue of what distinguishes regular man or woman (character), character developments, or character style (Millon) – from character problems.

A dearth of documented medical revel in concerning each the problems themselves and the application of diverse remedy modalities.

Numerous character problems are "now no longer in any other case specified" – a catchall, basket "category". Cultural bias is obvious in positive problems (together with the Antisocial and the Schizotypal). The emergence of dimensional options to the explicit method is mentioned withinside the DSM-IV-TR itself:

"An opportunity to the explicit method is the dimensional angle that Personality Disorders constitute maladaptive editions of character developments that merge imperceptibly into normality and into one another" (p.689).

The following issues – lengthy left out withinside the DSM – are probably to be tackled in destiny variants in addition to in cutting-edge research:

- The longitudinal path of the sickness(s) and their temporal balance from early youth onwards;
- The genetic and organic underpinnings of character sickness(s);
- The improvement of character psychopathology at some stage in youth and its emergence in formative years;
- The interactions among bodily fitness and sickness and character problems;
- The effectiveness of diverse treatments – communicate cures in addition to psychopharmacology.

All character problems are interrelated, at the least phenomenologically – aleven though we don't have any Grand Unifying Theory of Psychopathology. We do now no longer recognise whether or not there are – and what are – the mechanisms underlying intellectual problems. At best, intellectual fitness experts document signs and symptoms (as suggested via way of means of the affected person) and symptoms (as observed).

Then, they institution them into syndromes and, extra specifically, into problems. This is descriptive, now no longer explanatory science. Sure, there are some etiological theories around (psychoanalysis, to say the maximum famous) however all of them didn't offer a coherent, regular theoretical framework with predictive powers.

Patients affected by character problems have many stuff in common:

Most of them are insistent (besides the ones affected by the Schizoid or the Avoidant Personality Disorders). They call for remedy on a preferential and privileged basis. They bitch approximately severa signs and symptoms. They by no means obey the doctor or his remedy tips and instructions.

They regard themselves as unique, show a streak of grandiosity and a dwindled ability for empathy (the cappotential to realize and recognize the wishes and needs of different humans). They regard the doctor as not as good as them, alienate him the usage of umpteen strategies and bore him with their by no means-finishing self-preoccupation.

They are manipulative and exploitative due to the fact they consider no person and normally can't love or proportion. They are socially maladaptive and emotionally unstable.

Most character problems start off as issues in private improvement which top at some stage in formative years after which come to be character problems. They live on as enduring traits of the individual. Personality problems are solid and all-pervasive – now no longer episodic. They have an effect on maximum of the regions of functioning of the affected person: his career, his interpersonal relationships, his social functioning.

The regular sufferers is unhappy. He is depressed, suffers from auxiliary temper and tension problems. He does now no longer like himself, his man or woman, his (poor) functioning, or his (crippling) have an effect on on others. But his defences are so strong, that he's conscious best of the distress – and now no longer of the motives to it.

The affected person with a character sickness is liable to and susceptible to be afflicted by a bunch of different psychiatric issues. It is as aleven though his mental immunological machine has been disabled via way of means of his character sickness and he falls prey to different editions of intellectual illness. So a whole lot power is fed on via way of means of the sickness and via way of means of its corollaries (example: via way of means of obsessions-compulsions, or temper swings), that the affected person is rendered defenceless.

Patients with character problems are alloplastic of their defences. They have an outside locus of control. In different words: they generally tend in charge the out of doors global for his or her mishaps. In annoying situations, they are attempting to pre-empt a (actual or imaginary) threat, alternate the guidelines of the game, introduce new variables, or in any other case have an effect on the sector accessible to comply to their wishes. This is rather than autoplastic defences (inner locus of control) regular, for instance, of neurotics (who alternate their inner mental approaches in annoying situations).

The man or woman issues, behavioural deficits and emotional deficiencies and lability encountered via way of means of sufferers with character problems are, typically, ego-syntonic. This approach that the affected person does now no longer, at the whole, discover his character developments or behaviour objectionable, unacceptable, disagreeable, or alien to his self. As against that, neurotics are ego-dystonic: they do now no longer like who they're and the way they behave on a regular basis.

The character-disordered aren't psychotic. They don't have any

hallucinations, delusions or concept problems (besides
individuals who be afflicted by the Borderline Personality
Disorder and who revel in quick psychotic "microepisodes",
typically at some stage in remedy). They also are completely
oriented, with clean senses (sensorium), true reminiscence and
a excellent standard fund of knowledge.

The Diagnostic and Statistical Manual [American Psychiatric
Association. DSM-IV-TR, Washington, 2000] defines "character"
as: "...enduring styles of perceiving, bearing on to, and
considering the surroundings and oneself ... exhibited in a
extensive variety of essential social and private contexts."

The worldwide equal of the DSM is the ICD-10, Classification of
Mental and Behavioural Disorders, posted via way of means of
the World Health Organization in Geneva (1992).

Each character sickness has its very own shape of Narcissistic
Supply:

- HPD (Histrionic PD) – Sex, seduction, "conquests", flirtation,
romance, body-building, traumatic bodily regime;
- NPD (Narcissistic PD) – Adulation, admiration, attention,
being feared;
- BPD (Borderline PD) – The presence in their mate or partner
(they're fearful of abandonment);

- ASPD (Anti-Social PD) – Money, power, control, fun.

Borderlines, for instance, may be defined as narcissist with an awesome separation tension. They DO care deeply approximately now no longer hurting others (aleven though regularly they can't assist it) – however now no longer out of empathy. Theirs is a egocentric motivation to keep away from rejection. Borderlines depend upon different humans for emotional sustenance. A drug addict is not likely to choose up a combat together along with his pusher. But Borderlines additionally have poor impulse control, as do Antisocials. Hence their emotional lability, erratic behaviour, and the abuse they do heap on their nearest and dearest.

13.
Using Mind Control To Create An Addiction

With all of the paranoia of thoughts manage and the way Neuro Linguistic Probramming (NLP) may be (and is) used to "mess with peoples heads" it's excessive time to tug the cat out of the bag and allow humans understand precisely what's possible.

For example, are you able to create an dependancy in a person the usage of Neuro Linguistic Programming (NLP)?

Yes, you can.

Before you study the stairs to do it and the way to shield yourself, allow me provide you with warnings.

First, don't do that to humans except you're giving them a compulsion for some thing they need so that it will be accurate for them like exercize and healthful foods. Anything else and it could appear a laugh to consider however depart it at that. Only consider it, don't do it. It's simply now no longer a pleasant issue to do to humans.

Second, To do that you need to be superb at NLP, record constructing and anchoring etc.

Start with the aid of using eliciting what's referred to as the NLP submodalities of a compulsion someone has. You can do that with the aid of using asking what are a few matters they have got compulsions for, like chocolate, after which asking "As you experience that complusion what form of photos is your thoughts making? Where do you spot the ones pictures? How massive are the photos? Color or Black and White? " and so on.

Then start to describe what you need them to have a compulsion/dependancy for in precisely the equal way. Describe the brand new compulsion as being visible withinside the equal place, etc.

I'm now no longer going to offer you any extra element than that. It's extra than sufficient to test with.

Using this sample someone can create a compulsion for drugs, sex, money, perfection, riding fast, you call it, however you may additionally create compulsions for exercize, punctuality, orderlyness and plenty of so-referred to as "accurate" matters.

There are approaches to save you a person from covertly growing a compulsion in you. First be privy to the intellectual and emotional states that humans are asking you to explain and be on defend after they begin to speak approximately compulsions.

If you believe you studied a person has helped covertly create an undesirable compulsion in you (accurate luck) the compulsion may be undone with what's referred to as the meta yes/meta no process.

In Meta Yes/Meta No you'll begin with the aid of using deliberating some thing unrelated to the compulsion which you could say "No" to. Think of that object and convey up the very sturdy feeling and time and again say "No" in a completely company and congruent manner. Practice it till the "No!" and the sensation are deeply connected to at least one another. The subsequent step is to start saying "No!" time and again to the compulsion and do it with the equal power and conviction as whilst you began out the process.

14.
Personality Testing Myths And Realities

It is generally believed fable that persona trying out gadgets can degree your persona and are expecting your destiny behaviors. The pre-employment trying out mechanism has been following this creed with none strong evidence. The trying out enterprise claims all out validity. The academic establishments and organization corporations use them for screening purposes. Their transparency and fairness has even satisfied the courts of law.

But it's miles nevertheless an unresolved riddle; what do they take a look at?

Do they take a look at persona? What is persona then? What is its nature? How does it come into existence? Is it final results of evolution? Does count number has functionality to generate a persona? Why animals don't have a persona? Does it continue to be the equal all through complete of your life? And many extra questions.

It is like peeling off an onion. Every strip results in many extra. Finally you get a heap of onion strips. Where is the onion?

But personality isn't an onion...

Allport has recorded loads of various definitions. Most of the psychologists equate it on your style, behaviours and reactions.

They have devised gadgets to degree those important areas. The accrued records approximately your behaviours and temperaments assist them to determine your profession. You can also additionally arrange your behaviours in destiny however you can by no means be capable of pass for a profession of your passion.

Why?

Experts want to are expecting. They are expecting weather. They are expecting political situations. They are expecting financial conditions. They are expecting your destiny with signs, numbers, playing cards or palms. And they are expecting your destiny overall performance with the assist of personality trying out gadgets.

What's Your Personality?

It is nicely identified reality that each man or women has a personality. It isn't simply your bodily body. It isn't simply your consciousness. It isn't simply your ego. It isn't simply your behaviors. It isn't simply your bodily expression. It isn't simply your style. It isn't simply your temperament.

But all of them and plenty of different traits are expressions of your personality.

I don't locate it smart to outline persona. Admittedly it's miles an summary reality. You get it together along with your birth. You can both broaden it or disintegrate. Your style, behaviors and reactions are expressions of your evolved, undeveloped or under-evolved personality.

How do you look? How do you react? How do you talk? How do you live? How do you think? They all are expressions of your personality. The psychometrics measures those expressions and now no longer your personality.

The summary nature of personality can neither be measured nor be analyzed with any medical or non-medical tool. It can handiest be visualized. It may be evolved. It may be disintegrated. Your questioning and doing makes all out the difference. A evolved personality offers higher style, behaviours and reactions than an undeveloped one.

Why Psychometrics are Getting Popular?

The first actual motive is that each one desires to recognize who he is.

But larger motive in their big use is only a choice of the employers to keep away from bad-hire. They get loads of packages for a unmarried situation. They are the handiest to be had gear to keep away from idiosyncrasies.

They don't have options for psychometrics.

Tests are going to stay. Whether you are attempting to be admitted for a selected area or seeking out your dream job, you'll come upon psychometrics at one level or the others. You want to put together earlier than encountering them.

How to Prepare for Personality Testing Sessions?

Keep in mind... Personality is an great entity. You can think. You can visualize. You can discover. You can express. You can plan. You can create. You have limitless hidden potentials. But your preferred alternatives on paper are going to determine your destiny.

You must exercise offline and on line persona exams earlier than encountering a actual session. Your exercise shall now no longer handiest cause them to acquainted to you however additionally generate a listing of your strengths and weaknesses. You can enhance them together along with your aware effort.

However, it's miles an awful lot extra crucial to learn the way distinctive personality and flair exams degree expressions of your **persona**. What theories are **operating in the back of** them? How do they relate **distinctive** jobs with **distinctive** types? This **know-how** shall make it **lots simpler** to come upon psychometrics.

15.
Self Improvement And Success Go Hand In Hand More Than You Think

How do you realize if someone is inclined to gain self development? This is a query with out a precise answer. It will all rely upon the individual.

Many humans have goals, desires or targets however do now no longer realize the way to pass approximately attaining them. They can also additionally have notion approximately what could make up self development and their perfect lifestyles, however don't have any concept the way to even start to make the plans and take the moves required to cause them to a truth.

Some humans have a indistinct concept on the way to pass approximately self development. These are those that consider that if most effective that they'd a higher job, or have been given higher possibilities, or met the affection in their lifestyles, or something else, the entirety could be high-quality and they'd be satisfied.

They sense that their happiness or loss of happiness is determined with the aid of using outside elements and their mind and moves are of little consequence.

Some consider that if most effective that they'd extra cash they may have something they need and be on their manner to self development.

They can also additionally have spent little time considering what they truely need from lifestyles, and do now no longer genuinely consider there may be whatever they could do to create their fuzzy model of utopia anyway, aside from shopping for extra lottery tickets.

Other humans do now no longer even realize what they truely need from their lives and might actually have little concept what could genuinely makes them satisfied. They appear to simply flow from day to day, week to week, month to month, and 12 months to 12 months, and do little extra than pretty much get with the aid of using.

They can also additionally have reputedly stable jobs and be incomes sufficient to stay fantastically cushty lives. They appear satisfied sufficient and don't have any amazing ambition to acquire whatever extra from their lives than they presently have.

Is self development important?

The truth is that at some stage in our lives we're all continuously developing and developing. Circumstances make us develop and develop, although we do now no longer make the aware choice to do so.

Up to a positive age, we research via formal training and we keep to research via our reviews for the relaxation of our lives. We need to research and develop to address the entirety that lifestyles throws at us. We all need to undergo self development.

Modern lifestyles movements at a dramatically quicker tempo than at each time in history. For absolutely everyone dwelling in present day society there are extra possibilities to do whatever which you need to do together along with your lifestyles than ever before.

But there may be additionally extra opposition than ever before, and ever converting era method that there genuinely are few, if any 'jobs for lifestyles' anymore. It is now ordinary now no longer most effective to extrade jobs pretty frequently at some stage in our running lives, however even to absolutely extrade careers and industries.

Because the place of job is so competitive, individuals who are formidable and hungry for fulfillment realize they want to research new abilities and know-how to hold in advance of the pack. To gain this, self development is needed.

These are the humans a good way to be maximum probable to hold their jobs, or development inside their selected field, or a good way to be simply employable in exceptional corporations or industries.

A dedication to self development and private boom could be the finding out component in how absolutely everyone's destiny will flip out.

ABOUT THE AUTHOR

KANHA GUPTA is a professional Indian writer, web and graphic designer. He is a great digital artist. He is extremely fond of anything that is related to writing, digital design and all the yumminess attached to it. He's been freelancing for many years and now focuses on writing and blog design for small businesses and online publishers. He always aims to reach his creative goals one step at a time and believes in doing everything with a smile.

SOME IMPORTANT DIGITAL PRODUCTS

1) Natural Solutions For High Blood Pressure :-

https://291c9gfmwyh09td9p6n-vt2p63.hop.clickbank.net/

2) The Natural Way to Supercharge and Maintain A Healthy Brain & Vision :-

https://13c6f9dlszjxfl7olqplme0i1d.hop.clickbank.net/

3) 100 FITNESS AND HEALTH E-BOOKS :-

https://57c1d9eipyfy9z36kj27v9ry3w.hop.clickbank.net/

4) How I overcame anxiety disorder and started living life again :-

https://a176cjqdo2awfzc8xrwz5kgx0r.hop.clickbank.net/

5) Neuropathy No More :-

https://426ad9ccvzbshm4ps8zp2oieo7.hop.clickbank.net/

(Copy and Paste these links in any browser to avail them.)